HAPPY DIABETES

Being diabetic does not have

a disease, having diabetes is

a condition of life that you

can use as a benefit other

goals in your life

IMPORTANT NOTE: Before starting any sport or diet is essential to consult with your primary doctor or diabetes educator. This manual under any circumstances replace the concept or regularly visit and check a doctor.

INTRODUCTION

This manual that we developed with specialists in diabetes and under the experience will help you control your diabetes since psychologically and physically, normalizing their blood sugar levels in the blood, and therefore leading a healthy life and avoiding possible complications diabetes.

It is important to ongoing consultation with medical specialist and awareness that diabetes is a disease care, rigor and commitment to yourself.

We want to help improve their quality of life, and for that we have developed with dedication and rigor this manual, which should read carefully and regularly to achieve diabetes 10.

ATT

MillonMarketing.com

FIRST TOPIC

DM1 diabetes, insulin dependent or juvenile

WHAT IS DIABETES DM1, INSULIN DEPENDET OR JUVENILE?

Diabetes mellitus type 1 (DM1), known as insulin-dependent or juvenile, is an autoimmune disease that causes metabolic disorders due to the destruction of pancreatic beta cells responsible for insulin secretion. There is another diabetes, type 2 diabetes mellitus in which insulin does not the proper effect. It occurs in adults and does not always require treatment with insulin.

DM1 is characterized by an absolute deficiency in insulin secretion. This is a hypoglycemic peptide hormone, secreted in terms of blood glucose, and its main role in the body's glucose transport into cells.

As no insulin, glucose accumulates in the blood, resulting in hyperglycemia. This causes secondary pathophysiologic changes that generate long-term complications (retinopathy, neuropathy or nephropathy).

1.1 Clinical Manifestations

The clinical picture was characterized by hyperglycemia and the classic symptoms that can make us suspect a DM1 are:

• Intense thirst (polydipsia).

• Increased frequency of urination and urine (polyuria).

• Increased appetite (polyphagia), but with weight loss.

They can give other symptoms such as fatigue, nausea and vomiting, and ketosis ketonuria, glucosuria, and you can even get to diabetic coma.

1.2 Epidemiology

DM1 represents 5% of all types of diabetes, but children 95% of cases are Type 1 diabetes prevalence in Spain of 0.2% of the population, and an incidence of about 13 is calculated, 1 New cases per year per 100,000 inhabitants. The onset is most often placed during adolescence, with no differences by sex, but between 15-30 years there is a predominance of males. In any case differences in terms of socioeconomic status are observed.

1.3 Treatment: Insulin

Treating DM1 is a replacement therapy, which is given by the body insulin that he is not capable of producing. Insulin was discovered in 1921, and in 1923 the first solution of animal insulin (primarily swine) was marketed.

In the 80s, using techniques of biotechnology and recombinant human insulin synthesis, which changed the profile of action and reduce the adverse effects was obtained. Marketing first insulin analog was in 1996. Since 2001 commercial presentations are all in solution of insulin with 100 IU / ml; this certification has improved the decreasing dosage administration errors.

Insulins classes

A) According to the power and profile of action (start time and duration of effect):

• Ultra-fast action: start at 15 minutes; peak between 30 and 90 minutes; and up to 5 hours duration. They are insulin analogues (lispro, aspart and glulisine).

• Fast action: start at 30 minutes; maximum effect from 1.5 to 3.5 hours after the start; and maximum of eight hours. It is human insulin or Regular.

• Intermediate-acting: slower onset (1 hour); up to 4-12 hours; its effect covers 15 to 20 hours. They are the NPH insulin and lispro protamine.

• Long Action: Start from 1h; They have a basal profile without peak; and long-lasting (24h). They are insulin glargine and detemir.

B) Depending on its composition:

• Monocomponent insulins: formed by a single type of insulin.

• Bicomponent or biphasic insulins: fast or quick solutions protamine insulin intermediate-acting form.

Method of administration

The dosage of the insulin is variable as it has been adjusted to the needs of each patient; is so individualized treatment. The health care provider a pattern with the units of insulin to be administered in each situation. It is therefore important to know the glucose, which is measured with a glucometer, user-friendly device that measures blood glucose levels.

Instructions:

1. Wash hands with soap and water or your finger with alcohol, and let dry.

2. Place the strip into the meter.

3. Make a prick a finger with a new, sterile lancet and place a drop of blood, rejecting the first, on the test strip.

4. In a few seconds the blood glucose reading is obtained.

The route of administration is subcutaneous; but in special situations it can be administered intravenously, exclusively in hospitals. There are different areas where you can make the subcutaneous injection: Abdomen (separate two fingers navel and two fingers under the ribs), Arm (upper outer region), thighs (front and side area outside), buttocks (outer zone above).

Equally important is the injection switch and separate a pair of fingers each injection prior to avoid adverse effects in the area. We must also know that certain attitudes can vary the speed at which insulin is absorbed.

Devices for administration of insulin available are divided into:

• Pods: vials of insulin solution. The amount administered is extracted with a syringe, with which the patient will inject the dose.
• Multidose: pens preloaded with a reservoir of insulin solution; Simply select the dose on the device and proceed to the administration.
• Insulin pumps: devices for administering insulin infusion subcutaneously by a fixed catheter in the abdomen.

Insulins are kept in a refrigerator between 2 and 8 ° C, and once in use can be kept at room temperature (below 30), protected from direct light and heat for 28 days. Reject the past this time, or if they freeze or present lumps. It is also important to follow the instructions for use and conservation specified in the prospectus for each type of insulin and device.

Special precautions

Insulin, despite being a safe drug, can give an adverse effect:

• Lipodystrophy (so it is advisable to rotate the site of injection).

• Hypoglycemia (for mismanagement, excessive or poorly controlled dose).

Administration is contraindicated if there is intolerance to any of the excipients of the solution, and also in case of hypoglycemia.

Insulin may interact with different medications, which may alter blood glucose; the doctor will advise you to follow.

SECOND TOPIC

TYPE 2 DIABETES (DM2)

T2DM is also known as adult-onset diabetes, it is a chronic disease characterized by high levels of blood glucose (concentration of high blood sugar). Is a lesser known disease Diabetes Mellitus type I, in which the patient are required to take insulin through a puncture, to control blood glucose levels. T2DM, startup does not need insulin jab, but may need it if an early diagnosis is not made.

Specialists insist on early diagnosis of this disease, because in this way the patient may perform a less invasive treatment to solve their pathology, based on a balanced diet and physical activity controlled.

Mellitus Type II (T2DM) Diabetes has become one of the most serious health problems, as currently in the world the prevalence of T2DM reaches 12% of the population and one third of it know they have this disease is say, 4% of the population has T2DM and unknown.

What foods are counterproductive for type 2 diabetes?

• Dairy: Limit the fat and avoid all those carrying sugar, jams.

- Cereals: Cookies, pastries and brioche conventional.

- Vegetables: Those that are cooked with animal fat ingredients (sausage, blood sausage, bacon, etc.)

- Fruit: Fruit in syrup, dried fruit, candied and crystallized.

- Beverages: sugary juices, soft drinks with sugar, sugary milk shakes and alcoholic beverages.

- Fats: cream, butter, lard and tallow.

- Other: Chocolate and chocolate powder, honey and conventional jams, fruit jellies (lead sugar).

THIRD TOPIC

FOOD IN DIABETES

In diabetes it is important to maintain regular eating habits and make a balanced diet that will allow better control of the disease. Ideally make up to six daily meals avoiding intervals greater than four hours during the day fasting, and trying always perform at the same time to avoid sudden changes in blood glucose.

It is important to monitor to make a meal at mid-morning and mid-afternoon, as this is when insulin will make a greater impact and sugar can drop too low, causing hypoglycemia. You should know how many carbohydrates consumed at each meal. It is therefore important to know the glycemic index and the concept of serving. The glycemic index indicates the capacity of a foodstuff to increase blood glucose. Foods with a lower glycemic index are the most desirable (legumes, vegetables, pasta).

Simple carbohydrates: These are rapidly absorbed and rapidly increase blood sugar. Are glucose, fructose, lactose and sucrose found in fruits, honey, milk and table sugar. They are accompanied by fiber, fat or proteins, they are absorbed more slowly.

Complex carbohydrates: They are slowly absorbed. It includes glycogen, starch (found in vegetables, grains, beans and tubers), and fiber, the latter being indigestible.

The concept of a food ration relates to their carbohydrate content. A serving equals 10 grams of carbohydrates, and you have to know what weight of each food corresponds to a ration.

They are considered free foods or beverages, those that contain less than 20 calories and 5 grams of carbohydrates per serving.

FOURTH TOPIC

EXERCISE AND DIABETES

4.1 Introduction

Exercise is important for diabetics as it helps to control the disease, therefore should not be excluded from sports activities but you need to keep control. Exercise has the following effects:

• Increases glucose uptake in muscle.

• Increases insulin sensitivity.

• Lowers blood glucose concentration.

Exercise increases the risk of hypoglycemia, during practice and up to 18 hours later, especially in unusual intense exercise, as it increases insulin sensitivity. By this fact it is necessary to control your blood sugar and general rules to follow when exercising.

4.2 Before exercise

You have to make a measurement of blood glucose and act according to the value:

• 100-200 mg / dl Perform the exercise normally.

• 70-100 mg / dl Take carbohydrate foods before you start.

• <70 mg / dl or symptoms do not start exercising.

• > 250 mg / dl not exercise until normal values.

4.3 During the year

You should have easy access to a source of glucose or another carbohydrate that serve to treat or prevent hypoglycemia. In case of a long and intense exercise it is necessary to take a supplement of 10 to 15 grams of carbohydrate every half hour.

4.4 After exercise

You have to control your blood sugar to see if it needs to provide extra nourishment. The very long-term intense exercise can temporarily raise blood sugar, but then, by increasing insulin sensitivity, tends to lower and therefore no extra insulin in these situations is not necessary.

It is important to previously know the times that exercise is good practice to plan treatment. In case of an unusual or unforeseen exercise, and not being able to control blood sugar, take no food to prevent a possible hypoglycemia.

4.5 Exercise and Diabetes

Are well known negative effects, to health, it causes a lack of physical activity. Thus, sedentary lifestyle increases the risk of cardiovascular morbidity and mortality, but still an important risk factor for overall mortality. In addition, epidemiological studies clearly indicate a sedentary lifestyle as one of the major risk factors for developing type 2 diabetes.

The implementation of exercise programs for people with diabetes leads to these benefits when these programs are applied to the general population.

These benefits are basically:

- Reduced risk of cardiovascular disease

- Decreased blood pressure levels

- Increased levels of HDL

- Preventing Osteoporosis

- Increased self-esteem and other psychological benefits

- Increased energy expenditure and improved body composition

The practice of regular physical exercise provides additional benefits in the case of diabetes, particularly for patients with type 1 diabetes and 2. These benefits are basically a moderate improvement in glycemic control and increased insulin sensitivity.

4.6 The exercise in preventing diabetes

A sedentary lifestyle is directly associated with a higher risk of some metabolic diseases, including type 2 diabetes Regular physical exercise can help improve body composition, decrease resistance to insulin action and prevent DM2 development, especially in high risk populations, such as individuals with impaired glucose tolerance (IGT). Several studies have shown that therapeutic intervention physically active individuals have a lower incidence of type 2 diabetes compared to those sedentary.

Thus, the Finnish Diabetes Prevention Study included 522 individuals with IGT demonstrating a 58% reduction in the incidence of diabetes at three years of follow-up in this group made changes to their lifestyle (including moderate exercise). The Diabetes Prevention Program (DPP) observed in individuals with IGT 3234 reducing by 58% the risk of diabetes, this being more effective than metformin, which achieved a 31% reduction intervention.

4.7 Substrate energy exercise

In the practice of physical exercise, muscle glycogen is the main energy source for muscle contraction. This muscle glycogen is one form of storage of glucose in the body, comprising about 400g glucose (about 1500kcal) located throughout the body muscle mass. The body also has another reservation glucose as glycogen, localized in the liver, and with a storage capacity of more than 100g of glucose.

During muscular activity, the type of fuel used depends mainly on factors such as the intensity and duration of exercise. For gentle exercises, practiced mostly in low-intensity fat as energy substrate used. As exercise intensity increases also increases the rate of glucose used as an energy source.

According to the duration of the exercise, the first 30-60 minutes of muscular activity is mainly consumes glucose in their deposits in the form of muscle glycogen. When these deposits begin their depletion also started obtaining energy from circulating plasma glucose. It is at this point that other process begins hepatic glucose production, from molecules such as glycerol, lactic acid or some amino acids.

4.8 The hormonal response to exercise

These metabolic processes associated with the exercise are possible thanks to the participation of an efficient system that integrates nerve impulses with the hormonal response. The non-diabetic individual, physical exercise causes a nerve stimulation of adrenergic type, acting on pancreatic β cells by inhibiting the production of insulin.

This reduction in insulin levels did not affect the cellular uptake of glucose, since this exercise favors uptake similarly insulin. Thus, the decreased levels of circulating insulin allows increased hepatic glucose production by activating processes hepatic gluconeogenesis and glycogenolysis.

Another essential phenomenon is the stimulation of another pancreatic hormone, glucagon. This hormone is produced by the pancreatic alpha cells and is known to increase levels dramatically when blood insulin levels decrease.

Glucagon acts directly on metabolic pathways responsible hepatic glucose production, ie, glycogenolysis and gluconeogenesis. To this effect must be added the other group calls against regulating hormones, such as catecholamines, cortisol and growth hormone which also act on the liver leading to increased glucose production.

FIFTH TOPIC

COMPLICATIONS OF DIABETES

5.1 Hypoglycemia

Hypoglycemia is the most common acute complication. In a diabetic hypoglycemia is considered diminution in the blood glucose level below 70 mg / dl. This decrease in blood glucose can go with or without symptoms; when it appears provide a warning signal to start the treatment.

It usually occurs after excessive insulin or inadequate food intake, or after performing a higher exercise than usual without lowering your dose or taking a food supplement. The symptoms of hypoglycemia in the early stages are usually: hunger, headache, cold sweats, change of character, tremors and abdominal pain. In more advanced stages difficulty speaking or thinking, odd behavior, blurred vision, drowsiness and dizziness it appears. In severe cases it can reach altered consciousness, convulsions and coma.

Given these symptoms should be checked by capillary blood glucose, the existence of hypoglycemia. If you can not perform the test and there is suspected, it treats it like it is, and stop the activity being performed. In case of severe hypoglycemia should be treated with glucagon, a hormone produced in the pancreas, as well as insulin, but has the reverse function transforms liver glycogen stores into glucose, which is released in the blood, and the result of their effect is a rise in glucose values. It comes in a vial with the lyophilized glucagon and a syringe with sterile water.

To use:

1. Enter the water from the syringe into the vial and shake gently.

2. Remove the administered dose vial with the same syringe.

3. Administer by subcutaneous or intramuscular injection

To prevent hypoglycemia is important:

• Regularity in the amounts and timing of meals, administration of insulin and exercise; modify portions of carbohydrates and insulin doses in relation to exercise.

• Maintain proper administration technique, and with the right dose.

• Always carry a source of glucose, or sugar.

• Conduct frequent glucose self-analysis.

This makes it possible to decrease the frequency of hypoglycemia and treat them properly.

How to deal with hypoglycaemia:

1. If there is no alteration of consciousness:

• Initially ingest 10-15 grams of carbohydrates rapidly absorbed, like two lumps of sugar, fruit juice or regular soda (100 cc) or a glass of skim milk (200 cc). For immediate treatment they are not suitable whole fruit, whole milk or chocolate.

• After measuring blood sugar 10-15 minutes.

    - If you are not normalized: eat 10 to 15 grams of carbohydrates rapidly absorbed, and remeasure 15 minutes later.

    - If standardized: eat 10 grams of carbohydrates of slow absorption: 20 grams of bread, 3 cookies, a glass of whole milk, 2 natural yogurt or a piece of natural fruit.

• If hypoglycemia occurs close to a meal, a diet of fast absorbing carbohydrates will manage and advance lunch.

2. In case of severe hypoglycemia with impaired consciousness:

• Do not give food or solids or liquids.

• Administer a dose of glucagon intramuscularly or subcutaneously.

• Tell family, and go to the nearest emergency service. When the patient regains consciousness carbohydrates provide orally.

5.2 Hyperglycemia

It is the second most common complication occurring in diabetics, and is an increase in the blood glucose values above 250 mg / dl. It may be due to insufficient insulin dose by changes in diet, infection, trauma, stress, and / or states of dehydration.

When blood sugar is high, you may feel unwell with headache, drowsiness, excessive thirst and urination more often. In this situation, you should drink liquids without carbohydrates (the most appropriate drink is water), and may require administration of an extra dose of insulin. We must facilitate access to liquids and bath whenever they need. The hyperglycemia not become emergencies, but if a high value is checked to make routine checks of blood glucose, as if recurring may indicate decompensation.

SIXTH TOPIC

MODEL ATTITUDE FOR DIABETES

6.1 Diagnosing diabetes. Development and phase characteristics.

Diabetes is like having high blood pressure, epilepsy, asthma, Parkinson's or many other diseases called chronic, which currently can not be cured. Fortunately, given these conditions we have been able to develop highly effective treatments in most cases they have allowed the quality of life of affected people is getting better.

Despite these advances, which have facilitated the adaptation to the disorder, the fact is that the diagnosis of a chronic disease is a strong psychological impact on the individual and their family, and also has a negligible social consequences.

Obviously, the diagnosis of diabetes lead to changes in the lives of those affected. Having to follow a certain discipline of feeding schedules, measuring foods, take special care when exercising and take insulin, they are certainly compatible with normal life activities, but not always easy to carry out the changes involved. In any case, there will be time to adjust.

Family members should try to help those affected to live with the disease with the maximum comfort, trying to get on your skin and never denying the limitations. The diagnosis of a chronic disease affects the self-concept and triggers a series of defense mechanisms to protect against distress. This is a maturing process that every individual must pass when he has to face this new reality.

The process of adaptation to the disease develops in different phases. Not all people go through all phases, not always occur in the same order here will be exhibited, but more often than not do this.

The word "diabetes" can be lived in very different ways depending on the experience of the person concerned. Some people do not realize much of what it represents, while others are completely blocked because envision a future disabling, causing them obviously marked distress. During this stage it is difficult to think clearly. It is almost impossible to receive and understand the information that the professionals. Initially anxiety and low mood is generated.

Those affected at this stage, should find a receptive attitude in the professionals who should know ask and listen. The reaction of disbelief is almost constant passing to bad news. Sometimes, the initial reaction of disbelief still a passenger to become a true defense mechanism against anxiety phenomenon, and then we can talk about denial.

The affected person often downplay diabetes, ensuring that it does not create any problem or at other times saying: "I have no diabetes, only some sugar in the blood." In this effort of denial, the expressions of some people suggest that they try to convince themselves and convince the listener that having diabetes is better than having more.

During this phase, the affected people feel little involved in their disease and little motivated treated appropriately. "Why he has touched me?" is the most heard phrase in people who are at this stage. This feeling means that there are at least aware of the reality, but it does not want to accept. React with irritability, bitterness and disappointment can be natural at this stage. Self recalls the healthy person he was and the life seems unfair. Treatment is difficult, life has changed and you have negative or being different from others feelings.

The feeling of anger is common at this stage. Adolescents become especially difficult for healthcare professionals to famiialres revolt against the disease is added to the denial of any kind of standard; attitude, moreover, characteristic of this age, already critical. The voluntary withdrawal of one or more doses of insulin-nothing uncommon for the period- no longer a provocation and a desire to break the norm. Both parents and professionals should avoid confrontation. The understanding is as important as discipline.

It is mainly manifested by attempts to manipulate the treatment, "agreeing" some demands that are below the doctor suggests. For example: "Well, I have diabetes, but insulin put me"; or "Okay, I accept myself insulin but not more than once a day" In these cases there is full awareness of the disease. Although the patient, rather than rebelling in it negotiates with the hope of reducing the difficulties he perceives. Certainly not forget that there are a minimum of survival are not negotiable.

Remember that the family environment also passes through a phase of acceptance of the disease, which does not always coincide with rhythm and order in the affected person. Some prefer to simply call it adaptation; others think that adaptation would be a preliminary step to full acceptance. And finally, some say that we must "assume" the disease, not necessarily "accept".

In any case, it is understood that this phase is characterized by the encounter of emotional balance that allows serenely face treatment every day and their different social, family or personal implications. The information always becomes essential at this stage, very helpful.

The concepts of insulin, food self-analysis or assimilate and understand better. As mentioned before, not everyone will go through all the stages or remain the same amount of time, so that some diabetic fully accepted soon while others never come to assume. In those cases where it is anchored in a phase, a specific psychological help may be necessary. For example, if you are persistently in denial phase, the acquisition of knowledge for future living with diabetes will be prevented. The concentration of glucose in the blood, the condition of the retina or the driving speed of a nerve are relatively easy to measure parameters.

The mood and the degree of stress or anxiety are factors that must also be considered to better achieve behavior change. The importance of these factors on the control and stability of blood sugar are usually recognized by all, and experience teaches that when patients are concerned about a test or when you are under strong negative emotion -the separation the couple, the loss of a person rather estimada- diabetes suffers.

In recent times, there have been many studies showing that, with the same doctor treating people with a mood more stable, less prone to fluctuation and ability to confront problems, have better figures hemoglobin glicocilada and minor fluctuations in blood glucose than those with no such features.

6.2 Living with diabetes.

Diabetes carries a great deal of behavioral and emotional adaptation of the affected person. The experience of a child, youth or adult with diabetes in the family can vary depending on your age. It is natural that after diagnosis the family relationships are altered; therefore, in imposing standards of conduct we must distinguish those related to being a diabetic from those who are part of the education of the child or young person.

If every time you refuse or prohibit something done on behalf of the diabetes, the young man begins to reject the disease that so much grain. Especially if we also consider that many rules of conduct is subject the development of the individual and would apply even if not diabetic.

Therefore, it is desirable to standardize the sooner the relationship between parents and children and resume normal standards of behavior before diagnosis, referring diabetes as little as possible to the time limitations. If not provided bans diabetes will partner, when in fact many rules existed before that diabetes appeared.

Within the family environment, a factor that is associated with improvements in the control of diabetes is emotional communication. Family environment where members maintain emotional communication based on the fact externalize emotions, able to reduce the level of anxiety and promotes the adaptation of the affected person's disease.

Moreover, it is important to encourage the child, youth, adult or older to take an active approach in controlling diabetes person. For example, we must congratulate you when you have made the right choice in food or give a confidence when self-analysis is made or administer insulin. Also, it is important not to focus exclusively on the control of blood glucose, as this may create family tensions when results are not as expected.

Parents need support. You will find it in the health team and the association of diabetics, where they can share their experiences with others who have gone through a similar situation. The attitude of parents can help or hinder the process of acceptance and responsibility for the child or adolescent girl with diabetes. They described different types of parents or family attitudes that can influence the behavior and attitude of the young:

Perfectionist parents are those who want to control all aspects of treatment. They also tend to focus on what is not working well. The young man responds with rebellion, non-acceptance and rejection treatment.

Parents who are not involved at all in the treatment: to believe that diabetes care must follow the advice of professionals, without further implications. In these cases the child / youth often forgotten parts of the treatment on the grounds that to care just have to take insulin.

Protectionist parents believe that by having diabetes, must protect and take more care of his son. Do not let the young take steps in the treatment, and if it does and does not work, blame themselves immediately. Then, the young usually shows insecurity, adults need to do anything. Sometimes, you can try out performance of the disease or manipulate through this.

Parents shared responsibilities: Such parents teach learn from the disease itself. They give positive rewards when the guy does things correctly and allow them to learn from your mistake. In these cases the child usually shows up and autonomy.

Therefore, in the process of diabetes education should be considered not only as an educational subject the patient but also the family, in which you have to find the interlocutor.

6.3 Diabetes and friends

In many cases, such as diabetes and unseen to the naked eye, you choose to hide it. Hide the fact may indicate, sometimes, inadequate acceptance of illness or fear of not being accepted in the environment or reference group. It is logical that in the beginning there is some fear of communicating the disease in the environment.

This communication is possible when the person has already been adapted to treatment and provided, in the individual's history, there have been no previous experience of rejection of the sick person. However, the person should take the time to socialize the disease.

Apart from family, friends or desirable that the closest, school or work mates are informed about diabetes so they understand what is happening and what can help, especially in the case of hypoglycaemia.

www.ingramcontent.com/pod-product-compliance
Lightning Source LLC
Chambersburg PA
CBHW040926180526
45159CB00002BA/635